Resolving Complaints

FOR PROFESSIONALS IN HEALTH CARE

Wendy Leebov, Ed.D.

A Part of the Skills Development Series

Authors Choice Press

New York   Lincoln   Shanghai

Resolving Complaints for Professionals in Health Care

Authors Choice Press
an imprint of iUniverse, Inc.

For information address:
iUniverse, Inc.
2021 Pine Lake Road, Suite 100
Lincoln, NE 68512
www.iuniverse.com

Originally published by Mosby-Great Performance, Inc.

ISBN: 0-595-28361-6

Printed in the United States of America

ABOUT THE AUTHOR

Wendy Leebov is Associate Vice President of Human Resources of the Albert Einstein Healthcare Network in Philadelphia. She founded and was president of The Einstein Consulting Group, a nationally recognized health care consulting firm that helps health care providers improve service quality and employee performance. A dynamic trainer, speaker and consultant, Dr. Leebov has authored five books on customer relations, patient satisfaction, and service quality improvement for health care professionals. She has a doctorate in human development from the Harvard Graduate School of Education.

ABOUT THIS BOOK

In this book, we will discuss effective—and, in contrast, some not so effective—ways of handling customer complaints in the facilities and organizations dedicated to meeting people's health care needs, including nursing homes, hospitals, home care services, outpatient centers, physicians' offices and health insurance plans. Throughout, you will find examples of behavior representing effective and ineffective complaint management in familiar situations.

You will also find exercises that you can do to help you see both sides of typical complaint situations, to sensitize you to the customer's point of view, and to expand your own creativity and options for better meeting your customers' needs. This is your opportunity to become a complaint management professional!

OTHER TITLES IN THIS SERIES:

Assertiveness Skills
Customer Service
Job Satisfaction
Stress Management
Telephone Skills
Working Together

Complaints

Wouldn't it be great to work in a place where you never had to hear a customer complain? Or had to deal with an irate patient? Or had to respond to an impatient co-worker? Or needed to calm an angry family member?

That does sound nice, but it is not realistic. No matter how well organized, efficient and friendly a health care organization becomes, there will always be complaints. Sometimes these complaints will come from the patients or plan members. At other times they will come from patients' or plan members' families and friends. Complaints also come from physicians, physicians' staff, referral sources, insurance companies, utilization reviewers, and more. Still others come from your co-workers or your internal customers. All these people make up the primary customers whose needs you must meet every day.

Customer satisfaction is central to the success of any service organization, and yours is no exception. Excellent technical skills and medical expertise are, of course, the essential elements of the services your organization extends to the public. But today's health care consumers demand more. They want convenience, comfort, courtesy and respect as well as competent medical care. When one or more of these qualities is missing, the customer is likely to complain.

When things are going well, you rarely hear about it. People usually accept good service without comment. Even when things are not going well, you usually will not hear about your service problems. Studies have shown that more than 70 percent of the customers who are dissatisfied with an organization's services do not actually complain. They do not speak up about their dissatisfaction. Maybe they feel at your mercy and therefore they fear speaking up. Maybe they feel powerless and do not expect their complaint to do any good. Or, maybe they are just people who have difficulty being assertive. So, instead of complaining, they quietly go away mad and are likely

Customer satisfaction is central to the success of any service organization.

to take their future business elsewhere. What makes matters worse, these people who are dissatisfied but do not complain to you ultimately will complain to their families and friends, spreading your negative reputation. Consider these findings:

- A satisfied customer tells four other people about the care and service received from your organization.

- A dissatisfied customer tells 20 other people about a bad experience.

That means your organization has to satisfy five customers for every one customer it disappoints just to maintain its positive reputation.

A well-known principle in business, called the "10-10-10 Principle," states the problem clearly:

> *It takes $10,000 to get a customer.*
> *It takes 10 seconds to lose one.*
> *It takes 10 years for the problem to go away.*

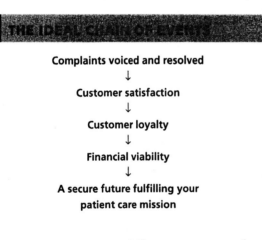

THE IDEAL CHAIN OF EVENTS

Complaints voiced and resolved
↓
Customer satisfaction
↓
Customer loyalty
↓
Financial viability
↓
A secure future fulfilling your patient care mission

The moral here is that every customer is essential to the well-being of your organization. The philosophy "you win some, you lose some" hurts your organization's effectiveness. Even though some dissatisfaction is inevitable, given the complex business you are in and the variety of people and personalities you serve, you can recover dissatisfied customers by becoming great at inviting, hearing and resolving their complaints.

When you are not hearing customer complaints, it does not mean that everything is OK. It may only mean that customers are quietly accepting conditions they dislike and planning never to return.

ENCOURAGING COMPLAINTS: THE PAYOFFS

The above statistics are bleak, unless you know how to turn dissatisfied customers into satisfied ones. How? By encouraging them to complain and by handling their complaints effectively. Dissatisfied customers are more likely to return to you in the future with their business if they voiced their complaint and you showed concern, understanding and, when possible, responsiveness.

People who do complain, people who speak up about their dissatisfaction, give you a second chance to make things right and to improve conditions, not only for a specific customer but for other customers who follow. When a customer points out a problem in your behavior or in your service, that customer provides you and your organization with the opportunity to make things better, to uphold and improve your reputation and standards.

The objective of complaint management, or service recovery, is first to recognize that there is a problem (to seek out the complaint) and then to identify the problem (to know what needs to be fixed) and to formulate a response (to do everything possible to fix it). The result will be a loyal following and a more efficient, respected organization.

Accrediting Agencies Care About Your Response to Complaints
Becoming aware of customer complaints is so important, in fact, that the Accreditation Manuals for hospitals and nursing homes put out by the Joint Commission on the Accreditation of Health Care Organizations now include specific guidelines for complaint management systems. Medical practices, home care services, ambulatory care centers, insurance companies, and medical care

organizations can learn a lesson from this and institute similar procedures to ensure responsiveness to their customers' complaints.

The Joint Commission requires that the following guidelines be incorporated into everyday procedures:

- A mechanism must exist for receiving and responding to complaints concerning quality of care and service.

- People served by the organization must be informed of their right to present complaints and the process by which they can present complaints.

- The organization must analyze the complaint and, when requested, take appropriate corrective action.

- Each customer making a significant complaint must receive a response from the organization that substantively addresses the complaint.

- If patients or their families are the complaining customers, the presentation of a complaint must not in itself serve to compromise any patient's future access to care or service.

SERVICE RECOVERY

Effective complaint handling

=

service recovery

=

turning lemons into lemonade.

The Fine Art of "Service Recovery"

Effective complaint resolution has recently earned a special name—service recovery. Service recovery means doing all you can to correct a wrong perceived by a customer so that the customer's interests are protected and his or her emotions calmed. The term "recovery" is used to reflect the need to help the customer recover—to restore them from a state of frustration or disappointment to a state of satisfaction.

Customers are impressed when you listen, apologize, acknowledge their inconvenience or discomfort, take ownership, provide alternatives, keep your promises, and do so in a timely and courteous fashion.

Service recovery experts talk about the need for an effective, responsive service organization to have a complete service recovery system that includes all of these elements:

- A system for inviting complaints.

- Staff with skills to listen nondefensively and sensitively when they first hear the complaint.

- Clear methods for directing complaints to the people with the power to do something about them.

- Allowable resolutions or things employees can do to solve or compensate for people's problems—without having to get their supervisor's approval.

- A system for tracking complaints, so the organization can identify patterns and do something to prevent them.

- A system for focusing on solving problems that are leading to repeated complaints.

People who speak up about their dissatisfaction give you a second chance to make things right.

5

WHAT'S YOUR ORGANIZATION'S COMPLAINT SYSTEM?

What do you know about your organization's policies and systems related to complaints?

- How does your organization invite customers to complain?

- Are there employees especially equipped to hear and respond to customer complaints, like a customer service, member services or patient relations department? If so, do you know how you can refer customers to them or call them yourself when you've heard a complaint?

- Is there a time frame within which you are supposed to respond to a complaint?

- Are there guidelines for how to respond to complaints (who to call, letters to use, etc.)?

- Are you required to document complaints of which you're aware and/or make anyone else aware of these complaints?

- Is there someone you, as a staff member, can call when you're stumped about what to do with a complaint you've heard?

If you don't know the answers to these questions, ask your supervisor so you can use every existing resource and system to help your customers or refer them to someone who can help.

MANAGING COMPLAINTS IS EVERYBODY'S JOB

No organization can control who the customer complains to initially. It may be a secretary, claims representative, billing clerk, technologist, physician, social worker, administrator, dietary worker, member of the maintenance or housekeeping staff, or a nurse. In any of these positions or in any other position in your organization, you may be the person a customer comes to first with a complaint. At that moment, you are the goodwill ambassador for your organization, with the responsibility to do whatever is needed to help the customer recover from his or her dissatisfaction. Your organization is counting on you to handle customer complaints professionally, compassionately, courteously and creatively.

Dissatisfied but uncomplaining patients tell family and friends, even their doctor, about their complaints.

As already mentioned, the vast majority of dissatisfied customers do not speak up when they have a complaint. Perhaps they are timid or fearful because they feel dependent on you and your organization—at your mercy. Or perhaps they have chosen just to put up with whatever happens until they can get out and go elsewhere. Read the stories that follow. They are typical of what happens with a dissatisfied but uncomplaining patient.

Hester Marmalade: A Hospital Fable

Community Memorial General Hospital launched an expensive advertising campaign. They flooded the media with powerful, attention-getting ads. People around the community started talking about Community Memorial General Hospital as a "place on the move." More and more, people requiring hospitalization asked their doctors whether they could go there.

Hester Marmalade was having stomach pains, and she was losing weight rapidly. Her doctor recommended hospitalization for an intense battery of tests. Ms. Marmalade, having been exposed to the media blitz by Community Memorial General Hospital, expressed her desire to go there for her tests. Her doctor agreed.

6

Ms. Marmalade arrived Tuesday at 8 a.m. The people in Admissions had told her that by arriving early, she could begin her tests immediately. That was fine with Ms. Marmalade!

However, because of delays in Admissions, Ms. Marmalade did not get to her room until 1 p.m. After settling in, she hoped the tests would start soon. A person in a white uniform stopped in and said she would be back shortly to get Ms. Marmalade ready for her first tests. Ms. Marmalade waited very patiently. And she waited. Ms. Marmalade was not annoyed, because being a very understanding person, she realized that hospital people are very busy with many patients.

She waited some more. That woman who said she would be right back—where was she? Ms. Marmalade waited. Getting nervous and wondering whether she had been forgotten, Ms. Marmalade pushed the call button. The woman who had been in much earlier poked her head around the door and said, in an intensely irritated voice, "I said I'd be with you in a minute!"

Ms. Marmalade cringed. She felt afraid.

In time, Ms. Marmalade had her tests done. She left the hospital and was relieved to know that she did not have cancer, as she had feared.

She went home and called her friends. After relaying her relief about the diagnosis, she went on to tell about the hospital worker who had spoken to her so harshly. It stuck in her mind. Ms. Marmalade told her friends and her doctor that Community Memorial General Hospital was not so hot, as hospitals go. In fact, she said, "I'll never go back to that place again!"

Each of her friends, sympathizing with their friend Hester, thought, "Neither will I."

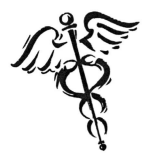

The story of Hester Marmalade demonstrates several sources of dissatisfaction common in health care settings. One source of dissatisfaction is being kept waiting for what seems excessive lengths of time without being told the length of or reason for the wait.

Another source of dissatisfaction is the feeling of being left isolated and ignored in an examining room or waiting area. Of course, there is the unnecessarily harsh and unpleasant response from the uniformed health care worker. Ms. Marmalade was possibly too timid or just not inclined to complain to representatives of the organization. Perhaps she did not know to whom she could complain. She certainly did complain to her doctor and friends. As a result, the hospital gained a negative reputation, undoing what had been the positive effects of the organization's advertising campaign extolling the virtues of the hospital to the community.

Mac Handy: A Health Plan Fable

Mac Handy is a member of Glenside HMO. He and his family leave town to visit their friends Mark and Lee, who live 100 miles away. While away, Mac offers to help Mark and Lee build a small addition to their friend's house. While working together, Mac drops some equipment on his foot, and Lee rushes him to the nearest hospital. Mac's foot is bleeding heavily and the bones feel broken. The hospital Emergency Department assures him that his health plan will cover his care and they provide Mac with the care he needs, telling him to call his health plan to report the incident right away.

Mac returns home after his trip and calls his HMO. He tells them that he is worried about getting bills for his care, since he was in an "out-of-plan" facility. His plan representative assures him that the hospital that cared for him will bill them directly and that he does not have to worry. They suggest further that, if he gets a bill, he should send it on to his health plan account representative. Two weeks later, bills start arriving, including bills from the Emergency Department, a physician, and a Radiology Service that X-rayed his foot. He sends the bills to his health plan representative with a reminder note about the situation. Two weeks later, he gets another bill from the hospital and calls his plan representative. She tells him that it takes them time to pay the bill, but that he does not have to worry about it—that they are taking care of it, and that he can tear up the second notice. He tears it up.

A month later, he gets another bill with a warning that, if he does not pay it, they will send it to their collection agency. Upset that this might interfere with his ability to obtain credit on a mortgage he has applied for, Mac calls his health plan and complains, "You said you would take care of it!" His plan representative says, "You have to understand that we're handling thousands of claims and that we will get to yours and handle it." When Mac asks "When?" his claims rep says "As soon as we possibly can!" Mac hangs up frustrated, annoyed, and worried about that mortgage. He thinks to himself: "What people say about HMOs is really true. They sell you on not having to worry about bills—that they'll take care of everything. Then, when the time comes, it's one hassle after another." Mac wonders "Maybe I should switch back to my old plan, or at least maybe I can find another HMO that gives better service."

Mac's story shows the critical importance of effective complaint management. Mac's plan rep reassured him that the problem would get solved, but apparently took no initiative to really resolve it. Also, this person did not tell Mac anything specific about how or when the problem would be resolved to Mac's benefit. Nor did he apologize for the hassle and inconvenience.

Each employee must do his or her part in making sure that the organization lives up to its public image. Advertising campaigns make promises, but only employees can keep them.

The stories of Hester Marmalade and Mac Handy show why each employee must do his or her part in making sure that the organization lives up to its public image. Advertising campaigns make promises, but only employees can keep them. That is why it is so important to sharpen your skills as a complaint management professional. We must assume the responsibility—and the challenge—of handling complaints responsively and competently.

9

ARE THERE COMPLAINT HORROR STORIES IN YOUR ORGANIZATION'S CLOSET?

Think about it. What customer complaints do you and your co-workers hear that you know are handled in ways that further disappoint your customers? Talk with your co-workers. For each horror story situation, consider:

■ **What situation is causing the complaint?**

■ **Put yourself in the customer's shoes. What does the customer feel and think about you and your organization when the complaint is handled inadequately?**

■ **What are the consequences of customers being made more unhappy by these situations?**

How Is YOUR Attitude Toward Complaints?

Imagine that a customer approaches you and says "I have a complaint." Of course, complaints do not always begin in such a simple and "civilized" manner. But imagine that is what just happened. What is your immediate, spontaneous reaction? Most people would probably think to themselves "Oh, no! Now what!" or "I sure don't have time to deal with this right now!"

Most people cringe when they sense a complaint coming. Most people, whether the complaint involves them directly or not, usually take complaints personally. However, it is exactly this kind of attitude that makes complaint handling so difficult and prompts employees handling complaints to become defensive and ineffective in the customer's eyes.

Sometimes when employees hear customer complaints, they unconsciously adopt the attitude that because the customer is already dissatisfied the customer is a "lost cause" and will never come back to the organization no matter how the employees respond. One research report suggests that this attitude is unfounded. Here are a few of the conclusions:

■ The average business never hears from 96 percent of its unhappy customers. In fact, for every complaint received, the average company has 24 customers who have had service problems, six of which are considered serious.

■ Complainers are actually more likely than noncomplainers to do business again with the organization that upset them, even when the problem isn't satisfactorily resolved.

■ When the problem is satisfactorily resolved, the instance of repeat business by a complainer zooms to 95 percent.

■ Customers who have complained and have had their complaints satisfactorily resolved will tell an average of five other people about the favorable treatment they received.

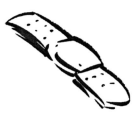

Source: "Customer Complaint Handling in America," Technical Assistance Research Program for the United States Office of Consumer Affairs, 1986.

The conclusion is clear. Even when a complaint is not resolved in the customer's favor, *the fact that someone listened to the complaint will greatly increase the likelihood of return business.*

That means we should not only be receptive to hearing complaints from our customers, we should even go about looking for them. In short, we should beg people to complain so that we can listen and, when possible, take action to make things right. That requires a positive attitude toward complaining customers (an attitude that is not always the first that comes to mind), a welcoming attitude.

Remember that in any service organization, customer satisfaction is a primary goal, and in health care it is a vital goal. We want customers to be happy with us, we want them to tell others that we are the best people to come to for health care services. We need to know what it is that we do that displeases them. We need to know so that we can address problems for them and for customers who follow them.

The next exercise will help you measure your attitude toward handling customers' complaints. Try this exercise again after you read this booklet and again after you have had one or more encounters with complaining customers and can put what you have learned to use.

Customers who have had their complaints satisfactorily resolved will tell an average of five other people about the favorable treatment they received.

Instructions: Recall three encounters you've had with an angry, complaining customer (a patient, a plan member, a physician, a co-worker—any customer). Pick instances that stand out in your mind. Think about the interaction and how you felt when you first realized that this customer had a complaint. Then answer the following questions.

SITUATION 1

■ *What was the situation?*

_____

_____

_____

■ *How did you feel when you realized the customer was voicing a complaint?*
   (Check all that apply.)

☐ Frightened?   ☐ Defensive?

☐ Angry?   ☐ Confident?

☐ In control?   ☐ Put upon or oppressed?

SITUATION 2

■ *What was the situation?*

_____

_____

_____

■ *How did you feel when you realized the customer was voicing a complaint?*
   (Check all that apply.)

☐ Frightened?   ☐ Defensive?

☐ Angry?   ☐ Confident?

☐ In control?   ☐ Put upon or oppressed?

SITUATION 3

■ *What was the situation?*

_____

_____

_____

12

■ *How did you feel when you realized the customer was voicing a complaint?*
(Check all that apply.)

☐ Frightened?　　　☐ Defensive?

☐ Angry?　　　　　☐ Confident?

☐ In control?　　　☐ Put upon or oppressed?

1. Looking at your feelings in response to the above three situations, how would you describe your overall attitude toward complaining customers?

_____

_____

2. Did you immediately understand the nature of the complaint? What was it?

_____

_____

3. Were you able to suggest or provide a solution? If so, what was it?

_____

_____

4. How do you think your customers felt when the interactions were completed?

☐ Satisfied?　　　☐ Appreciative?

☐ Dissatisfied?　　☐ Still angry?

5. How did you feel?

☐ Gratified that you could help?

☐ Frustrated because you couldn't help?

☐ Resentful for having been placed in this position?

☐ Unhappy with the customer who complained?

6. If you had these encounters to handle over again, what would you do differently?

_____

_____

_____

_____

_____

What Do Health Care Customers Want?

Customers approach a service organization because they want something, and very often what customers really want goes beyond the obvious. People come to your organization because they want health care services—that much is obvious. They want other things as well, things that are not as easily observable and that are just below the surface of their stated reasons for coming.

Psychologists have debated for years what it is that customers really want. After much study, 12 basic customer needs have emerged. When even one of these needs is not met, customers are likely to feel distressed and are more likely to complain. These basic needs are felt by health care customers as well as by consumers of other kinds of goods and services. Understanding these 12 needs will help you to interpret customers' complaints and to handle them with compassion and positive action.

Need #1: Customers Want Control Over Their Lives

The various customers of health care organizations and insurance plans all want control over their lives. This applies to customers needing health care services (patients in home care, ambulatory care, medical offices and hospital settings; health plan members; and nursing home residents) as well as to the covered family and friends of these people, and to customers who serve these people indirectly, such as insurance representatives, utilization reviewers, maintenance workers, administrators and many, many more.

Patients, health plan members and nursing home residents especially tend not to feel in control. Procedures are done to them, frequently without their active participation. They are often placed in situations where they feel helpless and at the mercy of others. To counteract this feeling, health care workers should try to help these especially vulnerable customers to feel that they are active parties in the decisions that affect their health and well-being. These customers also need to feel they are not being taken advantage of, manipulated or deceived. They need to feel that their consent is required and that

Health care customers need to feel that they are active, intelligent and respected participants in their own care.

14

their feelings and opinions matter. They need to feel that they are active, intelligent and respected participants in their own care.

The family and friends of people needing care also want to feel control and exercise it on behalf of their loved ones needing care. Family and friends will often speak up to caregivers to complain about what their loved ones feel they must "quietly endure." When a family member or friend speaks up with a complaint or a request on their loved one's behalf, that complaint or request must be treated with the same respect, courtesy and prompt action that it would receive if the patient, resident or plan member had voiced it.

Other people involved in health care delivery, but not with direct care, are also customers who seek control. When referral sources, claims reps, utilization reviewers, administrators, materials managers, quality monitors and others seek service from you, they want to know what they will get and when. They want to be able to count on you to provide what they need in order for them to do their jobs. If you keep them in the dark, they feel out of control and frustrated with your services. and they draw negative conclusions about the quality of the services you deliver to them.

Need #2: Customers Want to Achieve Goals

Customers need to feel that your services are helping them toward a goal. For example, when a physician customer is trying to locate a patient's chart and relevant laboratory results, he or she wants to feel that every interaction with a co-worker is moving him or her toward the goal of finding this important information. The same is true of your other customers. They want to know that what you are doing to them and for them serves an important purpose that will bring them satisfaction and help them achieve desired results. Customers respond negatively when they feel that the organization's activities are meaningless, needlessly time-consuming, or unrelated to their goals.

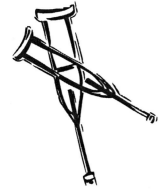

Need #3: Customers Want to Preserve Their Self-Esteem

Customers, like all of us, want to feel good about themselves no matter what they are doing. They want to think of themselves as intelligent, wise and competent. They do not want to think of themselves as silly, foolish or dumb. They will respond favorably to staff who support their self-esteem. In short, customers want to be treated with courtesy, dignity and respect. When this doesn't happen,

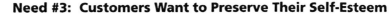

15

they respond with resentment, anger and, sometimes, rejection of your organization as a place fit to serve their needs.

Need #4: Customers Want to Be Treated Fairly

As is true in any business, health care customers want to feel that they are receiving the same attention, the same degree of competence, the same level of treatment, as everyone else you serve. Being treated fairly and appropriately is a basic customer need. In today's health care settings, treating everyone fairly is not easy, especially because different degrees and types of insurance support unequal levels of service for people. Too often, health care workers find themselves caught in a system where poorer people or people with inferior insurance receive inferior care, and this strikes these customers as unfair and inhumane.

Need #5: Customers Want a Friendly Reception

For the most part, customers come to your organization hoping and expecting to like and trust you and the other health care workers with whom they interact. They want those providing service to be friendly, warm and caring—and they want their service interactions to be as pleasant as possible. These are reasonable expectations and when they are not met, you can expect complaints—either to people within your organization or to friends and family later.

Need #6: Customers Want to Know What's Going On

Customers want to know what is happening and why. This is as true in receiving health care services as it is in buying a home or applying for a bank loan. Especially in health care, when one's body and overall well-being are the focus, a customer needs to know what (what tests, what procedures, what are my alternatives, what does it all cost) and why (why the tests are necessary, why the procedure must be done, and why the doctor has not seen them today).

People get frustrated and angry when they do not understand—or are not given enough information to understand—what is being done to them and why, the options they have, and the likely outcomes. That frustration can be compounded when the information they do get is given in such a technical manner, with jargon or initials, that they are left more confused than enlightened.

Need #7: Customers Want Security

Customers have a strong need to feel safe and secure. They want to feel physically safe, even protected, in the health care environment. They want your help in securing their belongings. They want their companions to be safe coming and going. They do not like unpleasant surprises. When their safety and security are at risk, they feel apprehensive and threatened. Unfortunately, their fear can easily turn into anger.

Need #8: Customers Want Approval, Acceptance and Recognition

Generally speaking, everyone needs the approval and acceptance of others, and this need affects our behavior in our role as customers. Health care customers are no different. Recognition is a powerful motivator. Customers want to feel that they are recognized as individuals who are important to you, that they are not just nameless faces with no more identity than their presenting complaints or diagnoses. Patients need to be made to feel welcome and accepted, and they need to be praised for their participation in their care.

Customers want to feel they are recognized as individuals who are important to you, not as nameless faces.

17

Need #9: Customers Want to Feel Important

All customers want to feel that they are important. They want those who interact with them to recognize their importance and not ignore them or treat them as bothers or interruptions. That means they expect full and prompt attention, and proper consideration.

Need #10: Customers Want to Be Appreciated

Customers like to feel appreciated. And well they should! If customers did not come to your organization, your organization would quickly fade out of existence, and you would not have a job. Customers deserve to know that their business—as well as their time, energy and trust—are valued and appreciated.

Need #11: Customers Want to Have a Sense of Belonging

Patients, physicians and health care workers alike prefer to identify with the organizations they patronize or work in. They want to feel that they belong, that they are insiders with a stake in the organization's success. This sense of belonging is aided immensely when employees remember customers and greet them by name, take the time to talk with them, respond to their complaints fully, and generally acknowledge the customers' loyalty.

Need #12: Customers Want Honesty

In the past, health care professionals were trusted without question and major business transactions were sealed with nothing more than a handshake. Today, however, the public is much more reluctant to trust businesses and other organizations. Americans, in general, are better informed than ever before about health care matters and the pitfalls of health care, and they need to believe that your organization and the people who represent it are honest and trustworthy. When patients or family members sense that facts are being misrepresented to them or that they are getting the runaround when they ask a question or that some dishonest dealing is going on, trust may not be the only casualty. Costly lawsuits and damaged reputations are real possibilities.

ARE YOU TYPICAL?

You just read a review of 12 needs of health care customers. To familiarize yourself with these a bit more, think of the last time you were a customer in a health care setting—a person in need of health care services. Review your experiences with the health care provider and ask yourself "How did the provider do in meeting these needs?"

	POOR	FAIR GOOD	EXCELLENT
Gave me feelings of control.			
Helped me achieve my goal in being here.			
Preserved my self-esteem.			
Treated me fairly.			
Gave me a friendly reception.			
Kept me informed about what was going on.			
Gave me a sense of security.			
Gave me approval, acceptance, and recognition.			
Made me feel important.			
Appreciated me.			
Helped me feel that I belonged.			
Was honest with me.			

Overall, how well did the provider do in meeting your needs?

SUMMARY OF CUSTOMERS' NEEDS

Customers consciously or unconsciously bring these basic needs into every interaction with your organization. Obviously, they do not come to your organization specifically to have these needs fulfilled. They come for health care services. To be completely satisfying, the services you and your organization extend should fulfill these needs. When you miss the mark, it's no wonder people complain.

WHAT DO COMPLAINING CUSTOMERS WANT?

We just reviewed what customers want in general. Now, let us look at what customers expect when they complain:

- **They want to be listened to.** This is a very basic need of complaining customers—to have someone listen to their complaints and acknowledge their feelings.

- **They want to be taken seriously and to be treated with respect.** That means responding to their complaints with sincere interest and concern. Customers do not want you to meet their complaints with sarcasm or offhand remarks like "You're kidding" or "There's no way that could have happened here."

- **They want immediate action.** When a customer has a complaint, he or she wants it taken care of now. Customers don't want to be put off until it's more convenient for you to handle the problem. They want you to respond immediately.

- **They want compensation.** Customers may want to be compensated financially for inconvenience, time lost or pain, or they may want a written apology from management or replacement of personal articles lost.

- **They want someone to be reprimanded or punished.** Of course, every complaint situation is different, but sometimes customers really want an employee in the organization to pay for what's happened to them. Sometimes a discreet report to your supervisor is appropriate if you believe the person responsible for the problem needs to be confronted by an authority figure. But often it's advisable to talk with your co-worker directly in hopes of notifying him or her of the complaint while there is

Complaining customers want to be taken seriously and treated with respect.

19

still time to do something positive about it. And customers want assurance that the people who, from their viewpoints, caused the complaint will get feedback about their dissatisfaction.

- **They want to clear up the problem so that it never happens again.** Sometimes making sure that it never happens again isn't entirely possible, but the customer will want to know that steps have been taken to correct the situation—even if it means correcting it only for future customers.

Not every complaining customer wants all of these things, but people would not complain if they did not want at least action or reaction. Although you will not always be able to meet every need for every complaining customer, you should be aware of these needs and do all you can to meet them.

The following exercise will help you examine your skills in meeting the dissatisfied customer's needs.

The customer may want to know that steps have been taken to correct the situation—even if it means correcting it only for future customers.

20

MEETING THE NEEDS OF COMPLAINING CUSTOMERS

Instructions: Recall an encounter you had with a complaining customer (a patient, co-worker, physician, caller to the organization). Pinpoint what the customer wanted and what you did or did not do to meet the customer's needs.

WHAT DID THE CUSTOMER WANT?	(CIRCLE ANSWER)		WHAT DID I DO TO MEET THIS NEED?
To be taken seriously and treated with respect.	Yes	No	
To know that immediate action would be taken.	Yes	No	
To receive financial compensation.	Yes	No	
To know that the employee responsible would be reprimanded.	Yes	No	
To be assured that the problem wouldn't happen again in the future.	Yes	No	
To have someone listen to the complaint attentively and with understanding.	Yes	No	

THERE ARE THREE TYPES OF DISSATISFIED CUSTOMERS

Not all of your customers will respond in the same way to distress, discomfort or an annoying problem. Some will be very open about their anger, but others will keep their feelings to themselves, and you may never even know they are dissatisfied. Still others, even though they are vocal about their discontent, will actually help you solve the problem.

There are three basic types of responders in anger-provoking situations: the passive responder, the problem solver, and the aggressive responder.

THE PASSIVE RESPONDER

Passive customers usually avoid the problem, keep their anger to themselves, and leave your organization never having told you of their discontent. As mentioned earlier, the passive responder can cause even more damage to your organization's reputation than the customer who voices complaints. The passive responder, like Hester Marmalade in our earlier fable, quietly goes away and often spreads bad news about your services to family and friends.

21

HELP PASSIVE RESPONDERS

Help passive responders open up with words like these: "I sense something's bothering you, Mr. Harper, and I really want to know what it is so I can try to do something about it. After all, I really want your experience here to be as positive as it can be. If you speak up, you'll give me a chance to understand and do something about what's bothering you."

Sometimes the passive complainer will hint at a problem without being explicit about its nature. "Here we go again!" or "What next?" are sometimes statements of discontent, and you should encourage the customer to explain further. Sometimes the passive complainer uses sarcasm to express discontent. For example, he or she might say "I hope I'm not keeping you awake" when the customer thinks an employee seems bored or disinterested in what is going on or being said.

When you let such signals of discontent go by unnoticed, you allow dissatisfied customers to damage your organization either by expressing their real discontent to their acquaintances or by not giving you the chance to identify problems and resolve them—for others as well as for this customer. The end result is that the organization loses customers and nobody really knows why. Also, whatever dissatisfied this customer will probably happen again.

Sometimes people adopt this passive approach to anger because as children they were taught that expressing anger is wrong and hurtful. As adults they simply keep their feelings to themselves. Other people do not speak up because they feel vulnerable—at your mercy—in the health care environment and do not want to risk making you angry with them.

It does not serve you or your organization to allow passive responders to leave without expressing their concern. That is why you should not only do your best to hear and resolve complaints, you should actually look for them. If you invite complaints in a manner that shows your sincerity, customers appreciate your openness and the time and effort you have devoted to finding out what went wrong.

The following adventure demonstrates a situation with a passive responder.

Resolving Complaints Adventure #1

Marty, a member of the maintenance team, had been working regularly in a nursing home and, with his outgoing personality, had gotten to know many of the residents. One morning Marty stopped into Mrs. Schubert's room to check the window seals. Mrs. Schubert was an elderly widow who had been living there for several months. Usually warm and talkative, that morning she seemed sullen and sad. She responded to Marty's greetings with one-word answers and an unsmiling face.

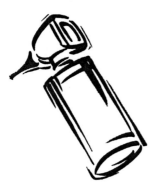

Marty could have accepted this and gone on with his work unconcerned. But he was concerned. Even though his work was more involved with tools and materials than with people and feelings, he cared about the residents he met.

"You seem a little sad today, Mrs. Schubert," Marty said. "Is there something wrong? Is there something you'd care to talk about? I'd like to be able to help if I can."

At first, Mrs. Schubert was a little shy about sharing her personal feelings. But Marty's concern seemed sincere, and eventually she got to the point. "I've been here for a long time now, and I haven't seen my grandchildren. I know I'd feel better if I could spend even half an hour with them. But they tell me the children are too little to come here to visit me."

Marty had no children of his own, but he was the uncle of three nephews and nieces. He knew how small children could light up one's life. But he also knew that the area of the nursing home in which Mrs. Schubert lived did not allow children under 12 years old to visit residents in their rooms. Sympathetically, he explained the reason behind the policy to Mrs. Schubert, but he knew that there was no real answer to her problem. Then he had an idea.

"Mrs. Schubert," he said thoughtfully, "I know children aren't allowed in this part of our facility, but I've noticed that the nurses sometimes take you to other parts of the home in a wheelchair. I'm going to talk to Lee Palmer, your unit manager, and see whether we can somehow arrange to have you visit with your grandchildren in an area outside your room. Would that make you feel better?"

If you invite complaints in a manner that shows your sincerity, customers appreciate your openness and effort in finding out what went wrong.

Outcome: 23

In fact it was possible, although not routine, to take the very sick Mrs. Schubert by wheelchair to a lounge, where she spent time on more than one occasion with her grandchildren. The visits helped to raise her spirits.

Mrs. Schubert did not forget Marty. Lee Palmer, the unit manager, was also grateful to him for his friendliness and thoughtfulness. She had also noticed Mrs. Schubert's decline in mood and was glad that Marty had taken the initiative to get to the root of the problem.

At first a passive complainer, Mrs. Schubert was resigned to suffer in silence. But because of one worker's interest and perceptive intervention, she ended up feeling good about her new home and about the caring employees who worked there.

THE PROBLEM SOLVER

The second type of responder, the problem solver, is easier to deal with than the passive responder. Problem-solving customers feel that it's OK to express their anger in positive ways. They may be emotional, but they maintain control of their emotions. They are assertive, and they take an active role in trying to find solutions to their problems.

The problem solver may say something like "I am very angry about the way I've been treated, and I would like this situation resolved." The problem solver tells you up front that something is wrong and gives you a good opening for starting to resolve the problem. These customers expect a prompt and efficient problem-solving response and are likely to be patient and cooperative when you resolve the issue quickly.

Such customers are very important to your organization because they point out problems, breakdowns, hassles and frustrations that otherwise might be overlooked by people in your organization. They offer you valuable opportunities to make things right and to improve the organization for everyone.

Resolving Complaints Adventure #2

Mae Willis is an advice nurse in a large HMO. She received a call from a member named Mark Waxman. Apparently Mr. Waxman called Appointments to arrange for a doctor or nurse practitioner to see his daughter who had a high fever and was throwing up. He failed to get a timely appointment and called the advice nurse number. Mae Willis answered.

Mr. Waxman explained: "I'm very frustrated with this situation. My daughter is very sick and I can't get a quick appointment. She's had strep throat before and I don't want to wait until someone has an opening. I want someone to get a throat culture and I want it today. I don't want the situation to get worse. I'm not satisfied when your colleagues tell me that the first appointment is tomorrow!"

Mae Willis apologized and said she could understand Mr. Waxman's frustration. She repeated that the flu season had all caregivers swamped with sick children. Mr. Waxman said: "That may be, but I pay my premiums and I want someone to see my daughter today. I can come in right away or any time today. I'm willing to have her seen by any competent person, not just the people she usually sees. Or you can approve a referral to a place that will see her!"

A "problem-solver," Mr. Waxman started out angry, but proceeded to suggest several ways to address his complaint. He was focused on the

The problem solver tells you up front that something is wrong and gives you a good opening for starting to resolve the problem.

24

goal of getting his daughter seen and he was willing to help solve the problem.

THE AGGRESSIVE RESPONDER

Some people are instantly angry because it is their style, or because whatever happened to them was so hurtful that it incited their anger. They express it through an aggressive response. As the word aggressive implies, this type of responder is likely to express frustration and hostility. At the extreme, aggressive responders may become verbally or even physically abusive. Often they lose sight of their real goal—to get their problems resolved—and become intent on getting even. They may launch a verbal attack against someone, but after they have let off steam, they often calm down and allow their anger to subside. As their emotions quiet down, these complainers sometimes feel guilty or embarrassed by their own behavior.

Some aggressive responders are people who learned early in life that the way to make people do what you want is to throw a tantrum. Hostile and aggressive expressions of anger can be learned responses built up over many years.

Resolving Complaints Adventure #3

Lucille Hankin lives in New York and came to visit her mother in Philadelphia after her mother arrived home from a long hospital stay. Lucille had spoken with the hospital social worker to arrange for a home health aide to stop in every morning to give her mother a bath, change her dressings, and make sure she was eating.

Although her mother assured Lucille on the phone that everything was fine, Lucille decided to visit to see with her own eyes how her mother was doing. She made the trip to Philadelphia to visit. To her chagrin, she found her mother with a bloody, soiled bandage and no liquids or food nearby. When she asked her mother whether the home health aide had been there, her mother said "No, not since two days ago."

Lucille was furious. She called the agency and demanded to talk with someone in charge. She yelled: "How can you stay in business? You're irresponsible and you're killing my mother! I'm reporting you to the authorities and I'll do everything I can to get your license taken away."

The social worker tried to get a word in that her mother had called to suspend home care, but Lucille was not listening and, eventually, hung up the phone with a bang.

Lucille responded aggressively. She would not listen, and she threatened the social worker. And the problem did not get solved.

Problem solvers may respond aggressively, too, if you do not respond to them promptly and positively. Responding aggressively may be a last resort in dealing with built-up frustration and resentment. Almost anyone might strike out in a hostile and aggressive manner when anger is allowed to build without outlet or relief. Again, that is why we should dig for complaints, so that a customer's anger never has the chance to reach this level. It is why we should take care to respond to problem-solving types as quickly and as efficiently as possible. Even the most reasonable, rational, helpful customers can be driven to aggression when their complaints are not adequately addressed.

SUMMARY OF DISSATISFIED CUSTOMER TYPES

The three types of complaining customers are seen in health care organizations every day. The expression of a complaint rarely means that the organization or an employee is totally wrong. Usually it means that something is wrong—one thing or a few things—but it need not result in a complete rejection of the organization as a whole. The point is that you, as a key representative of your organization, need to fine-tune your skills so that you can respond effectively to this variety of customers.

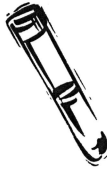

PITFALLS TO AVOID IN RESOLVING COMPLAINTS

There are many pitfalls to look out for in your behavior when resolving complaining customers. See if you can identify with any of the most typical pitfalls:

■ **Becoming defensive.** Very often, when someone complains to us, even when the complaint doesn't affect us directly, we take it personally. Comments such as "I only work here" or "It's not my fault" tend to turn customers off immediately. Defensive statements like these only make the situation worse. Do your best to remain objective, open-minded and flexible. Do not judge or act superior. Do not verbally attack the complainer. Instead, try to make them feel good about themselves. If you find this too difficult to do at the time, say nothing—do not say something negative that might offend the customer.

- **Citing organization policy.** Very often health care workers think it's a personal obligation to uphold organization policy, even at the expense of customer satisfaction. "I'm sorry, but that's the way we do things here" or "It's our policy" are neither productive nor creative responses to a customer's problem. Sometimes it's possible to give the customer at least one option that does not violate organization procedures if you get creative in a tough situation. Other times you might be able to bend rules when you know you're acting in your organization's best interest. When the rule really can't be avoided or bent, you can almost always help the customer anyway by listening and sympathetically explaining why the rule exists.

- **Poor listening.** When you fail to listen adequately to customers' complaints—when you interrupt them, act unconcerned, or minimize the complaints—you will almost always increase their hostility. Listen to what customers are telling you. Fix your attention on your customer. Nod, look concerned, and do all you can to absorb the feeling and content of their message so that they will feel listened to and so that you can respond effectively.

- **Giving the runaround.** Passing the buck, telling the customer to see your supervisor, or saying that there's nothing you can do about the complaint or that you're too busy to look into it will also promote the customer's frustration and alienate him or her further. Don't shift responsibility unless there is a specific policy for handling complaints, and then only after you have listened to the complaint and have explained how it will be handled under the policy.

- **Nonverbal behavior.** Sometimes the things we don't say speak louder than the things we do say. Looking annoyed, fidgeting, appearing rushed, avoiding eye contact, continuing to attend to paperwork—all these nonverbal behaviors turn customers off, make them feel unimportant, and aggravate the problem. These

Defensive statements only make the situation worse. Do your best to remain objective, open-minded and flexible.

27

behaviors, although they sometimes emerge "naturally," make the customer feel that what he or she has to say is of little or no importance to you or to the organization. Respond verbally and pleasantly to complaints.

- **Overreacting.** Since you want to resolve the complaint to the satisfaction of the customer and to the satisfaction of the organization, don't offer hasty solutions to the problem or make promises you can't keep. Sometimes it's sufficient for customers just to let off steam and voice their complaints. In some cases you need only to put customers at ease and help them regain emotional control.

- **Siding against the organization.** The customer may have some strong complaints about your services that even you think are valid. However, it really doesn't serve your purpose or the purpose of your organization for you to side with the patient or make remarks such as "We get complaints like this all the time" or "Sometimes I wonder whether this place knows what it's doing myself." Unfortunate events can occur even in the best-run service, and one customer's complaint is no reason to condemn the entire operation. Also, when a complaining customer is interacting with you, you are your organization's ambassador of goodwill. If you condemn your organization, you make your organization and yourself look bad, and you undermine the customer's confidence in ever using your services again.

When we are faced with a complaining customer, these actions are nonproductive and only reinforce the notion that the organization is unresponsive, uncaring, and not a place of choice for obtaining needed health care services. Take a moment to review the list of pitfalls and think about times when one or more describe your reaction to an irate customer. Most of these behaviors arise from being made to feel uncomfortable in a situation where you may not be at fault at all. You may have felt caught between wanting to help this customer and wanting to uphold the policies of your organization. You may have felt—perhaps justifiably—that the customer's complaint was unwarranted and that you really could do nothing about it. Or you may very well have been too busy at the moment to pay attention or to resolve the situation.

It is of urgent and immediate importance to listen and pay attention to the person who has a complaint, even when you're very busy.

28

The challenge is to put yourself in the customer's position. The customer feels very strongly about a problem and needs to talk to you about it. You have probably been in a situation when you complained to a store or a service organization and did not receive the attention or courtesy you felt you were due. How did you feel? Would you have felt better about that business if someone had at least given you proper attention, even if they could not resolve the problem immediately and perfectly?

Above all, it is of immediate importance to listen and pay attention to the person who has a complaint, even when you are very busy. Sometimes, after listening, you may need to refer the customer to your supervisor, to an administrator, to a patient representative, or to someone else in a better position to do something about the problem. But listen first and find out what the problem is, allow the customer to defuse his or her anger, and courteously and respectfully let the customer know what you intend to do about the problem.

DO YOU AVOID THE PITFALLS?

Figure out which co-workers are in a position to overhear you when you deal with complaining customers. Ask these people to give you feedback about the extent to which you avoid the pitfalls many people fall into when they handle complaints.

HOW OFTEN DO YOU:	NEVER	RARELY	FAIRLY OFTEN	VERY OFTEN
Become defensive	1	2	3	4
Cite organization policy as a reason to say "no"	1	2	3	4
Listen poorly	1	2	3	4
Give the customer the runaround	1	2	3	4
Give off negative nonverbal signals	1	2	3	4
Overreact	1	2	3	4
Side against the organization, undermining the customer's confidence in it	1	2	3	4
TOTAL				

Suggestions?

Handling Complaints Adventure #4

Mr. Riley, a businessman who knows the value of being on time, arrived 10 minutes early for his 9:00 a.m. appointment with his cardiologist, Dr. Rhodes, and took a seat in the waiting room. This was his first visit to Dr. Rhodes, and he was scheduled to be the first appointment of the day. As he sat, time passed and other patients started filling the empty chairs.

At 9:30, Mr. Riley still had not been called. By that time he was fidgeting nervously in his seat, glancing frequently at his watch, and quietly becoming more and more angry.

At 9:40, impatient and uncomfortable, Mr. Riley stood up and walked to the reception desk. "I hope I'm not inconveniencing anyone," he said sarcastically to the three people behind the desk, "but I had a 9:00 appointment. I made it three weeks ago. My time is very valuable, and I've already been kept waiting for 40 minutes. Where is Dr. Rhodes?"

The three people behind the desk—Karen, the department secretary; Anne, the nurse; and Steve, the blood technician—stopped what they were doing and looked at Mr. Riley. Karen, the person closest to him, spoke up, although any one of them could have spoken first.

Which of the following responses do you think she made to handle this complaint effectively?

1. "This is a very busy department, and you can't expect Dr. Rhodes to see you the minute you walk in the door! I'm sorry, but you'll just have to wait."

   Wrong: This is a defensive response that does nothing to relieve the customer's anger or to correct the problem. Mr. Riley was given no information to help him endure his wait in better spirits. If he did sit back down rather than leave in a huff, his anger would only have continued to build. His time, after all, is valuable.

A helpful response is not defensive and includes both empathy and information intended to explain the source of the problem.

2. "Mr. Riley, I know you were here on time, and I'm very sorry that you've had to wait this long. Dr. Rhodes had a serious emergency to attend to at 8:00 this morning, and that has put her behind schedule. I'll call her right now and find out how much longer you'll have to wait. Then you can decide whether you want to continue to wait or whether you'd rather reschedule."

Better: This response is not defensive and includes both empathy and information intended to explain the source of the problem. (Note that this information must be factual—in this case, Dr. Rhodes did indeed have an emergency that morning. It also includes a "plan of action"—calling the doctor for more information—and a choice of possible outcomes—staying or rescheduling.)

In the second case, Mr. Riley very likely felt he was getting the attention and concern he deserved. His anger was defused by Karen's sympathetic reply, as well as by having a reasonable explanation for the delay. When Karen called Dr. Rhodes and learned that the doctor would be ready to see Mr. Riley in 15 minutes, Mr. Riley was relieved to see an end to his waiting and agreed to stay for the examination. The problem was resolved.

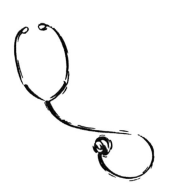

The Steps in Skillful Resolving of Complaints

The good news is that you can become much more skillful in resolving complaints if you learn, practice and apply the following 10-step process. This 10-step process is a sure way to help your customers recover from dissatisfaction to a state of satisfaction or even delight when they realize how caring and responsive you have been.

STEP 1: LISTEN WITHOUT INTERRUPTION

Customers with complaints may be timid and passive, open about their anger and rational, or hostile and aggressive. In any case, the first thing to do is to hear out their complaints. Put aside whatever you are doing and focus your complete attention on the customer. When a customer is ranting and raving, allow him or her to express all of his or her emotions without interruption. When you listen to the complaint, this phase usually passes, the aggression subsides, and you can deal rationally with the person and the situation.

When customers are timid and shy, you will need to draw them out so that you can listen. Maintain eye contact and use phrases such as "I can see this is very difficult for you" or "Please go on; I really want to hear more about this."

Also, you may need to be careful to protect the customer's privacy. If the customer is in a public area, within hearing distance of other people, suggest moving to a private area where you can communicate confidentially.

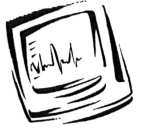

Write down vital information, and read each important point back to the customer to show that you have listened and to be sure you have gotten it right. You may need to convey the complaint to someone else in a position to help, and you will want to know that you have all the background information needed to correct the problem.

Ask questions. When people are emotional, they may not think to express all the details you might need in order to follow up on the problem. If you do not understand certain aspects of the patient's complaint, ask for clarification.

When you listen to the complaint, aggression subsides, and you can deal rationally with the person and the situation.

HOW WELL DO YOU LISTEN?

Do you find yourself planning what you're going to say next while the customer is still talking?	Yes	No
Do you find your mind wandering?	Yes	No
Do you think you know what the customer's going to say and stop listening?	Yes	No
Do you have trouble shifting your attention away from what you were doing and onto this customer?	Yes	No
Next time you listen to a customer complaint, repeat back to the customer your understanding of what they said, before you proceed to respond.		

33

STEP 2: DON'T GET DEFENSIVE

Even when the complaint is about your own behavior, it's important not to become defensive. Just because you've done something that a customer interprets as displeasing, it doesn't mean you are a bad person or even that they think you are. Similarly, a complaint about the organization's systems or other personnel need not be taken as a reflection on you. To do so would get in the way of effective and efficient complaint handling.

You can show your concern without having to agree or disagree about the facts of the situation.

Don't add fuel to the fire by disagreeing, arguing, fighting back or losing control of yourself. That would only compound the problem. Maintain your composure, stay calm, and try to slow the interaction. Be aware of the customer's facial expressions and body language, and plan your interaction accordingly. Remember that when you welcome the complaint and listen without interruption, the customer probably will gradually calm down and become able to discuss the problem much more rationally.

Sometimes, of course, the tirade may go on and on. Apparently the customer wants to be absolutely sure you have understood. It helps, then, to show that you have understood and to try to move the interaction to the stage of problem solving. Consider a well-stated request such as this: "Let me make sure I've thoroughly understood the problem here. Then we can discuss how to go about solving it. Is that OK? Here's my understanding of the problem…" Such a statement shows that you grasp the problem at hand and helps to bring the customer's focus back to possible solutions and actions.

DO YOU SHOW DEFENSIVENESS SIGNS?		
Do you feel like the customer is insulting you?	Yes	No
Do you disagree quickly with what the customer is saying?	Yes	No
Do you find yourself arguing with the customer?	Yes	No
Do you fight back and say something negative to the customer about their own behavior?	Yes	No
Do you ever lose control of your own behavior in response to a customer complaint?	Yes	No
If you answered yes to even one of these questions, consider taking a workshop on listening, assertiveness or complaint handling, so you can learn to hear complaints without taking them personally and getting defensive.		

STEP 3: USE A "SAD BUT GLAD" STATEMENT

"I'm sorry there is a problem, but I'm very glad you're bringing it to our attention. That gives us an opportunity to help you." Such simple statements serve several purposes. First, they let the customer know that you care about his or her dissatisfaction. They also demonstrate your recognition and appreciation that the customer spoke up and pointed out a deficiency. The customer knows that you care not only about his or her dissatisfaction but also about the feelings of all your customers. Such statements convey an open-minded attitude of the entire organization toward righting wrongs and ensuring customer satisfaction.

Apologies are effective when used appropriately. When you say "I'm really sorry you've been frustrated" you show your concern without having to agree or disagree about the facts of the situation. Then you have time to look into the facts before admitting blame. However, when a complaint is directed toward something you may have done or neglected to do, a simple personal apology may be in order. Otherwise, listen carefully and empathetically to the complaint before responding.

"Sad but Glad" Practice

For each of the following situations, write a "sad but glad" statement that will show your regret at the customer's disappointment, while appreciating the customer for speaking up.

SITUATION   "SAD BUT GLAD" STATEMENT

Example:

Patient was kept waiting.

"I'm very sorry we've kept you waiting, and I'm glad you called it to my attention so I can look into the delay."

Member felt rushed by the doctor.

_____

_____

_____

_____

_____

Billing person was pushy to a patient with financial hardship.

_____

_____

_____

_____

_____

A doctor was angry because the specialist did not call him to discuss a decision about his patient.

_____

_____

_____

_____

_____

STEP 4: EXPRESS EMPATHY

Empathy is the ability to feel a situation from another person's point of view. To use a familiar expression, empathy is putting yourself in the other person's shoes. Empathy is very important in complaint management, both in identifying with the customer's problem and in defusing emotions.

Show that you understand the customer's feelings with statements such as: "I can imagine how that must have been very frustrating for you. I can understand how angry and upset you feel about this." It helps the customer to feel understood and not alone in feeling frustrated and angry. It also opens lines of communication that help the customer calm down and willingly help to resolve the problem. A variety of responses to complaints are offered below.

Verbal Responses to Customers' Complaints

Defensive Responses: Defensive responses should be avoided at all costs, even when you're tired, busy or occupied with other thoughts. For example:

- "It isn't my fault!"

- "That's not my job!"

- "You can't possibly be right about this!"

- "Our organization would never do such a thing!"

- "Why are you telling me this? I wasn't there!"

Helpful Responses:

- "You seem upset. Please tell me more..."

- "Perhaps I've misunderstood. Can you please explain that to me again?"

- "I'm glad you brought this to my attention. I'd like to look into it."

- "If I understand correctly, you're saying that..."

Empathy opens lines of communication that help the customer calm down and willingly help resolve the problem.

Empathetic Responses:

- "I can appreciate how you're feeling about this."

- "I can see how upsetting this is to you."

- "It certainly sounds as though we've caused you some inconvenience."

- "I know I'd be upset too, if that happened to me."

Thanks for Complaining:

- "Thank you for speaking up about this. It gives us the chance to fix it and make sure it doesn't happen again."

- "Thanks for taking the time to tell us about this. If you hadn't, we might never have known about it."

- "Thank you for pointing this problem out to us. I'll be sure it's taken care of as quickly as possible."

Empathy Practice

List below the three complaints you hear most frequently. Next to each, write an empathetic statement that acknowledges the feeling that the typical customer communicates in the situation.

COMMON COMPLAINT   TYPICAL CUSTOMER FEELING/EMPATHETIC STATEMENT

1. _____

_____

_____

2. _____

_____

_____

3. _____

_____

_____

STEP 5: ASK QUESTIONS TO CLARIFY THE PROBLEM

Angry people sometimes distort the facts. After customers have had time to calm down, the information they offer may be different from the information they gave when they first expressed their complaints. Specifically, anger can lead to exaggeration. When emotions are quieted, summarize the facts as you understand them so far. Put into your own words what you have heard the customer say. Then ask questions to fill in the exact details of the events. Repeat the information back to the customer to make sure that you have it right. You both should agree on what the problem is. Then you can start considering how to resolve the problem.

When emotions are quieted, summarize the facts as you understand them so far. Then ask questions to fill in the exact details of the events.

Pinpointing with Questions

In the preceding exercise, you identified three common complaints you hear in your job. For each of those complaints, list below the questions you can ask to clarify the details of the problem, so that you can respond more effectively.

39

SITUATION	QUESTIONS I COULD ASK TO CLARIFY THE DETAILS
1.	
2.	
3.	

STEP 6: FIND OUT WHAT THE CUSTOMER WANTS

Even when customers complain about specific problems (for example, "My dinner was cold" or "The doctor disregarded the medical records I brought him"), don't jump to conclusions about what they need to feel better about the situation. The obvious solution does not work in every situation (for example, offering another dinner or mentioning the patient's complaint to the doctor). Sometimes the only outcome complaining customers want is a promise that you'll relay their complaints to the responsible parties. Sometimes, when their complaints reflect frustration about an unavoidable fact of life in health care, all that is possible is for you to listen with understanding and explain as best you can.

Occasionally, the customer will ask for an outcome you are not able to ensure. In such cases, you will have to relay the information to someone else who can take appropriate action or find someone who can (the supervisor, the social worker, or the patient representative). Thank the customer for the information, show that you are taking it seriously and, without sounding like you are passing the buck, explain that you will personally bring the complaint immediately to your supervisor or administrator or to someone else who can help. Once you have done this, do not let the matter drop. Check back with the customer and let him or her know you have followed through on your promise and, if possible, what is going to be done about it.

Finding Options

Consider the three situations you identified earlier. In each situation, the customer probably has a desired resolution in mind. What question can you ask to find that out? Also, find out what options are available to you in these typical situations, so you have some options to offer the customer!

	QUESTION TO FIND OUT CUSTOMER'S PREFERENCES	OPTIONS I CAN OFFER THE CUSTOMER
SITUATION 1		
SITUATION 2		
SITUATION 3		

41

Check back with the customer and let him or her know you've followed through on your promise.

STEP 7: EXPLAIN WHAT YOU CAN AND CAN NOT DO

Very often, customers in a state of distress or anger do not know or even care whether they are complaining to a person who can actually do something about their problem. You may receive the complaint because you were the only person in the area at the time a customer decided to complain, or perhaps because the customer thought you had an authoritative or approachable look about you.

There are times, of course, when you can handle the complaint directly and do something positive about it. Before you make any promises to the customer, explain what you can and can not do. If the customer wants you to do something beyond your power, offer to carry the ball—to locate the right person and represent the patient's concern to that person. The customer should only have to complain once. Then the person hearing the complaint should stay involved until actions are taken and the customer is made aware of the result.

Get specific.
Let the customer
know who will do
what, when, why
and how.

What Can You Do? What Can't You Do?

In each of the above situations, there are probably some actions you can take and some that you can't take, because they're too costly, or you don't have the authority to do so, or for another reason. It's important to think through the limits and opportunities.

For each of your common complaint situations named earlier, what options can't you offer the customer? And what options can you offer the customer? Press yourself to think of alternatives.

	I CAN'T...	I CAN...
SITUATION 1		
SITUATION 2		
SITUATION 3		

STEP 8: DISCUSS THE ALTERNATIVES FULLY

The customer may request an outcome that is not only impossible for you to deliver but is also unrealistic or impossible for the organization to deliver. While the customer is with you, discuss all alternative courses of action that you think could, in any way, address the problem. Because most alternatives have drawbacks as well as benefits, ask the customer to choose the option he or she prefers. Give the customer that power. Then get specific. Let the customer know who will do what, when, why and how. The customer will know that you are serious about helping.

If you have described the options and the customer is not satisfied with any of them, you may conclude there is nothing further you can do. In that case, offer to take the complaint to a higher authority.

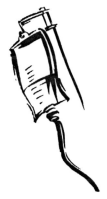

Discussing the Alternatives
So that the customer can choose the option that suits him or her best, you'll need to describe them fully. For each of your three complaint situations, describe fully below two options you can offer, including the details of "what, when, where and who."

SITUATION 1 *(Option 1)*

_____

_____

(Option 2)

_____

_____

SITUATION 2 *(Option 1)*

_____

(Option 2)

_____

SITUATION 3 *(Option 1)*

_____

(Option 2)

_____

43

STEP 9: TAKE ACTION

By now you have agreed on a course of action and it's time to take steps toward implementing the solution. Act promptly and keep your promises. Notify your customer regularly of your progress, and tell him or her immediately and honestly when a new plan of action must be pursued.

Taking Action

Most people intend to take action to follow up on a customer's complaint, but things get in the way. What obstacles do you face after promising to take action on a customer's complaint? Below are typical obstacles. How can you overcome each obstacle?

OBSTACLE	I CAN OVERCOME THIS BY...
I forget what I said I'd do.	
I can't find the right people.	
I get distracted by other people and tasks.	
I just don't have time.	
I rely on other people whom I can't necessarily trust.	
Other?	

STEP 10: FOLLOW UP TO ENSURE CUSTOMER SATISFACTION

Once the complaint has been resolved, it is important to follow up with the customer to make sure the solution was helpful. At this time, thank the customer again for bringing the problem to your attention so that you had a chance to make it right. You can also say something like: "I hope this problem won't happen again. I know I'll try very hard to see that it doesn't."

It's important to follow up with the customer to make sure the solution was helpful.

Follow-Up

For your three common complaints, what do you need to follow up on? Also, how can you make sure the customer knows you followed up?

IMPORTANT FOLLOW-UP...   I CAN BE SURE THE CUSTOMER KNOWS BY...

SITUATION 1

_____

_____

_____

_____

SITUATION 2

_____

_____

_____

_____

SITUATION 3

_____

_____

_____

Now, use what you have learned in the next exercise.

USING EFFECTIVE LANGUAGE

Instructions: To be effective with these 10 steps, you need to find effective language. In a staff meeting, training session, or lunch with a friend, help each other develop the "ideal" language in response to the following situations:

1. A nursing home resident complains to a nurse: "The lighting in here is awful! How can a person read?"

_____

_____

_____

_____

_____

2. A customer in a physicians' office complex complains to a receptionist: "I made this appointment weeks in advance! I said then that my time is valuable and that I needed to be seen on time. I've been waiting patiently for over an hour, but now I'm losing patience."

_____

_____

_____

_____

_____

3. A medical office staff member calls a hospital's admissions office to set a surgery appointment for a patient. She says, "This is Helen in Dr. Pike's office. I called three hours ago about getting a bed assignment for Hal Smith, and I haven't heard a word. Are you people on vacation, hard of hearing, or what?"

_____

_____

_____

_____

_____

Before you actually take steps to refer a complaint to someone else, consider carefully who would be the best person to address the complaint.

WHEN TO REFER COMPLAINTS TO SOMEONE ELSE

When resolving a complaint is beyond your authority or professional expertise, you may need to consult someone in higher authority or refer the complaint to your organization's complaint specialist. Unfortunately, customers may interpret this as passing the buck or brushing them off. The language you use is very important to avoid giving this impression. For instance: "I want to make sure we do all we can to respond to your concern and because of that, I want to involve (name). She(he) is our (job title) and is in a good position to help."

Before you actually take steps to refer a complaint to someone else, consider carefully who would be the best person to address the complaint. If you are not sure, ask your supervisor.

Here are important steps to follow when referring a complaint to a colleague in a better position to address it:

- Have all the facts about the problem on hand. Be sure you have confirmed all information with your customer and have recorded the relevant details.

- Have a clear idea of what the customer wants you or your organization to do about the problem.

- Relate your interaction with the customer to the appropriate person. Explain the alternatives you offered and the benefits and drawbacks you discussed. Be accurate and honest. It won't help the situation if you are more concerned with looking good than with resolving the customer's problems.

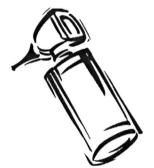

- If you made any promises to the customer, tell your colleague about them. Since you heard the customer's complaint directly, offer your recommendations as to what might be done.

- When you turn your information over to your colleague, make sure you agree on what role, if any, you will continue to play in the resolution of the problem or in keeping the customer informed. Ask to be informed of progress so you can be sure that the complaint was eventually resolved and the customer was told the result.

When Do You Need to Refer a Complaint?

Name three complaints that you should appropriately refer to someone else. Next to each, write down a very positive statement you can use to communicate this to your customer.

COMPLAINTS I NEED TO REFER   HOW I CAN TELL THE CUSTOMER WELL

1. _____

_____

_____

_____

2. _____

_____

_____

_____

3. _____

_____

_____

_____

TO DOCUMENT OR NOT TO DOCUMENT

Your organization needs to keep track of complaints received from customers not only because the accrediting agencies that oversee your facility may require it, but also because your organization needs to identify repeated complaints—patterns—that deserve attention and prevention-oriented problem solving. If you are not aware of how your organization tracks customer complaints, ask your supervisor. If he or she does not know either, use the sample format provided below and send it to the administrator or customer relations specialist responsible for setting priorities for problem solving and service improvement.

Sample Format for Documenting Complaints

1. The customer's name.

2. How to contact them (address, room number, phone number).

3. Background on the situation (time, place, people involved, event).

4. How the customer defined the problem.

5. How you responded and/or options you described.

6. What you promised or agreed to do.

7. Any suggestions you have regarding the solution.

8. How you can be reached for questions or a report on results (your name, position, phone number, address).

Are Telephone Complaints Special?

Not all customer complaints take place face to face. In a typical health care organization, hundreds of complaints are voiced over the telephone daily. The task of dealing with these complaints falls to the people who answer the telephones. If you receive telephone complaints, you know that those who answer the calls are rarely directly responsible for the original problem, even though some callers may not seem to realize that. Because the impression callers receive from telephone interactions colors their impression of the entire organization, it is essential that people who routinely take telephone calls become expert at handling complaints in a professional manner.

The principles for handling complaints by telephone are very much like those discussed previously. When handling complaints—or any other transaction—by telephone, the caller does not have the benefit of seeing your facial expression or body language or having eye contact. That's why it's so important to convey your interest and concern by your tone of voice, inflections and choice of words.

49

When handling complaints by telephone, it's important to convey your interest and concern by your tone of voice and choice of words.

Here are a few tips that can help you handle telephone complaints and keep your organization's reputation for caring intact at the same time:

- Give the caller your undivided attention, and express your sincere concern.

- Allow the speaker to have his or her say. Don't interrupt.

- Write down all important details, including short phrases and major facts. Don't be afraid to ask questions so that you have the correct information.

- Repeat these facts back to the caller to be sure you have understood and recorded them accurately.

- Be sympathetic, not defensive; this helps to calm the caller.

- Maintain a pleasant and even tone of voice. Don't lose your cool!

- Tell the caller exactly what you intend to do about the complaint you've received, to whose attention you will bring it, and when a response can be expected.

- Apologize to the caller for the inconvenience or difficulty even when it's not your fault or the fault of the organization. This is an important gesture of goodwill toward the public (for example, "I'm really sorry you've been inconvenienced").

- Thank the caller for bringing the difficulty to your attention and giving the organization an opportunity to make it right.

- Be sure to follow through with any action you promise.

Don't be afraid to ask questions so that you have the correct information.

MAKE SURE YOU ARE CLEAR ON THE GROUND RULES

Very often, customers' complaints are direct and straightforward, and you can resolve them yourself with little difficulty. For example, if a nursing home resident complained that her lunch tray was late, you could call Dietary Services and ask that a tray be sent immediately. Or if a clinic patient complains that he has been waiting too long to see the doctor, an apology, an honest explanation, and a revised time estimate would help to calm the customer.

Sometimes, however, complaints are more complex or more difficult for you to handle. You should clarify your own boundaries or latitude to act. Ask your supervisor what you are able to do for a customer without being out of line and, perhaps, bending the rules of the organization beyond their breaking point.

In a customer-oriented health care organization with a priority on customer satisfaction, you should be able to discuss these guidelines with your supervisor.

ASK YOUR SUPERVISOR...

- How much freedom do I have to bend rules to satisfy a complaining customer? Under what circumstances would it be OK for me to act without permission?

- How should I respond when money or special resources are needed in order to satisfy the customer? Suppose a patient prefers a certain type of pillow for sleeping and we don't have it. Can I go out and buy one and be reimbursed? If so, what permission do I need to do such a thing?

- Suppose the cooperation of other people or departments is required to solve a problem. What channels do I need to go through to get that cooperation? I certainly want to follow through quickly for the sake of the customer, but at what point is the solution out of my realm?

- To whom do I go when I don't know what to do about a complaint? Who would be the correct person to contact to get the answers I need as quickly as possible?

- Under what circumstances am I required to tell my supervisor about a problem or complaint? Would that be only when I can't solve it myself?

- When am I expected to document a complaint, and how do I go about doing that? Is there a special procedure for this?

- When is a written response to a complaint appropriate? Who actually writes the response, and what should such a response look like?

- When I hear the same complaints over and over from many people, and the problem is beyond my ability or authority to solve or prevent, where can I take this problem so that I, my co-workers, and the organization can fix it at its root and prevent future dissatisfaction?

The more freedom and power each individual worker has in resolving complaints, the more efficient complaint management becomes for the organization. You will find that there are areas in which you do not need to ask permission to act, and your ability to act independently speeds the resolution process and lessens the customer's resentment at being shuffled around. It also proves to the customer that the organization has faith and confidence in your ability to make responsible and effective choices.

Summary

It is so important that the complaining customer be treated with respect, courtesy and responsiveness that some key elements of complaint handling bear repeating:

- Listen patiently to the customer's complaint without interrupting. Don't argue or become defensive; allow the person to vent his or her emotions.

- Accept and acknowledge the customer's point of view, frustration or inconvenience. Show empathy. Consider how you would feel if you were in the customer's shoes.

- Ask questions to understand the problem fully and what the customer wants. Don't jump to conclusions about how the problem should be resolved.

- Fully discuss alternate solutions and options. Explain clearly what you can and can not do.

- Reach closure. Don't leave the person hanging. If you can't resolve the problem yourself, find someone who can, and tell the customer you'll get back to him or her. Arrange a time and method for communicating the results.

- Genuinely thank the person for speaking up, and explain why you are grateful that he or she pointed out a shortcoming. For example, you might say "It gives us a chance to make things right" or "Your feedback helps us to improve our service" or "We want to do right by you and you've given us a second chance."

- Follow through. Do what you said you would do, when you said you would do it. Keep your promises.

- Document the complaint according to your organization's guidelines.

Complaint management is everyone's responsibility. Handling complaints effectively from the start benefits everyone involved, and it helps to keep small complaints from becoming big ones.

Handling complaints effectively from the start helps to keep small complaints from becoming big ones.

53

0-595-28361-6

9 780595 283613